Clinton's Specialist Quota

Shaky Premises, Questionable Consequences

David Dranove and William D. White

T0273127

The AEI Press

Publisher for the American Enterprise Institute

WASHINGTON, D.C.

1994

ISBN 9780-84477-024-6

THE AEI PRESS
Publisher for the American Enterprise Institute
1150 17th Street, N.W., Washington, D.C. 20036

Printed in the United States of America

Contents

In legislation pending before Congress, the Clinton administration proposes to increase substantially government regulation of entry and training of physicians in the United States. The president proposes to create a National Council of Graduate Medical Education (NCGME) within the Department of Health and Human Services. The NCGME would oversee medical residency training programs. In section 3012 of the legislation, the NCGME is charged with ensuring that "of the class of training participants entering eligible programs for academic year 1998–1999 or any subsequent academic year, the percentage of such class that completes eligible programs in primary health care is not less than 55 percent." Moreover, the NCGME shall have the authority to "make allocations among eligible programs of the annual number of specialty positions that the Council has designated." Such allocations will be made to achieve geographic, racial, and ethnic diversity in training.

Restrictions of this kind and magnitude are unprecedented in medicine or, indeed, in any other profession we know. The federal government has historically provided extensive subsidies for pre- and postgraduate medical education. But it has never had a major role in directing specialty training. In a single step, the Clinton plan would delegate control of both the type and the location of specialty training to the executive branch of the federal government and would mandate dramatic changes in the training distribution of American physicians.

Two basic premises underlie Clinton's proposals for specialty quotas. The first is that a major imbalance has developed in the distribution of primary care physicians and specialists in American medicine, resulting in unduly costly and fragmented care. The second is that market forces will not address this imbalance, necessitating massive government intervention in medical education, with quotas as the policy of choice. Both premises are problematic for the following reasons:

- Specialization is a powerful mechanism for increasing quality and productivity in virtually all activities. It results from increases in the demand for skills, and it is a sign of a healthy, prosperous economy. Specialization in medicine in the United States brings with it unpar-

1

alleled quality and has provided a highly effective framework for the rapid diffusion of new technological advances.

- Skeptics argue that quality improvements in medicine have come at an unnecessarily high cost and fragmentation of care. They attribute high costs and fragmentation to the proliferation of specialists. But the problem is not simply specialist proliferation. At the heart of the problem is technological change—the former makes no sense without the latter. Underlying the debate about specialists is a far more significant, and as yet unresolved, debate about how we address technological change and who receives what kind of care.

- How purchasing of medical care is organized plays a key role in determining the use of specialists and technology. A central thrust of managed care is to restructure the way care is bought, to rationalize the use of new technologies and specialists. If managed care organizations demand fewer specialists and more primary care providers, market forces will accomplish what the advocates of quotas seek to achieve by fiat.

- If the demand for specialists does not decrease under managed care, then the result of the specialist quota will be either (1) a shortage of specialists with resulting nonprice rationing; or (2) a substitution of physicians or nonphysician providers specializing in particular activities but lacking formal specialty credentials. Either result would be undesirable.

- Continued strong demand for specialists under managed care may indicate either that (1) the appropriate demand for specialists is greater than believed by advocates of the quota, or (2) managed care organizations have been unable to rationalize the use of specialists. If (1) is correct, quotas could have dangerous consequences. If (2) is correct, it is almost certainly symptomatic of a broad failure of managed care, and this failure brings into question the entire Clinton health reform strategy. Specialty quotas are unlikely to remedy such a failure.

- The legacy of government intervention in medical manpower supply is not encouraging to those who advocate its expansion. If the past is prologue, then the Clinton quota will lead rapidly to an oversupply of primary care practitioners and shortages in selected specialties, particularly in emerging specialties.

- To the extent that government efforts are desirable to guide the production of specialists, quotas are a blunt and highly risky instrument to address what is fundamentally a problem with medical technology. Other more flexible types of strategies are available to the federal government and should be considered first. Federal subsidies of residency training, which cost taxpayers more than $5 billion annually, are prime candidates for cutbacks. Other strategies include reexamining federal payment policies for reimbursing health care providers, removing limitations on the use of nonphysician providers, and removing geographic barriers to mobility associated with licensing laws.

- Specialization may be symptomatic of a far more serious source of medical cost inflation: the development and extensive use of new diagnostic and treatment modalities. If managed care is unable to address this, then the most important direction for government action is to reevaluate its role as a central funder of research and development in the health care field.

This monograph establishes each of these propositions. The following section offers a critique of the arguments given by quota supporters. The next section provides a general framework for understanding the policy issues associated with the growing supply of specialists. We offer a market-based explanation for the growth of specialists. Against this background, we then consider in the ensuing section some of the possible inefficiencies that critics have argued may be associated with specialty proliferation. This provides a basis for considering the implications of capping the supply of specialists. An important issue that we take up in the subsequent section is the distinction between specialization as a functional and as an organizational phenomenon. In the next section we review the rather sobering history of federal manpower policy in medicine. The next section ponders the implications of specialty caps for the organization of medical care delivery, in the context of continuing technological change. We conclude with several specific recommendations for Congress to consider as alternatives to the Clinton proposals for specialty caps.

Rationales for Regulating the Supply of Specialists

The basis for arguing that there is an imbalance between the numbers of generalists and the numbers of specialists, which must be solved through government intervention, is fourfold. First, the ratio of specialists to generalists is far higher in the United States than in other countries, and it is increasing. Moreover, specialists earn far higher incomes than do generalists. Second, the widespread use of specialists unnecessarily increases costs. Third, the use of specialists does not improve quality. Last, America is waking up to a "new style" of medical practice, known as managed care, which is oriented more toward primary care and therefore requires more generalists and fewer specialists. While there is evidence consistent with most of these claims, the extent to which it supports the conclusion is controversial.

Too Many Specialists, Making Too Much Money. Specialists account for about 70 percent of all active physicians in the U.S.[1] This is an all-time high, having increased from 67 percent in the mid-1980s.[2] In Western Europe and Canada, specialists account for only 30 to 50 percent of all physicians.[3] At the same time, U.S. specialists earn substantially higher incomes than do generalists.[4] Physicians in specialties such as cardiovascular medicine, otolaryngology, orthopedic surgery, and radiology earn, on average, more than $250,000 per year, net of expenses. Physicians in general–family practice and general internal medicine average under $150,000 per year.

In important respects, it is not surprising that the United States has a greater supply of specialists than have most other industrialized nations. The United States far outspends other nations for medical care. Greater expenditures imply a bigger market for care, which in turn implies more opportunities for specialization. Critics respond that expenditures are excessive in the United States because there are so many specialists.[5] To evaluate this "chicken or egg" problem fully, we must weigh the role of payment systems and expectations regarding access to technology. Most other industrialized nations directly or indirectly cap demand for costly technology through global budgets for health care. Reduced use of specialists and their technological arsenals should be viewed as a result of these budget constraints; the converse seems improbable.

Nor are high wages for specialists in relation to generalists surprising, if specialization requires significant capital investments and special abilities. It would in fact be surprising if there were not differences. More to the point are questions about whether returns to specialty training are disproportionately high in relation to the necessary investments and effort, that is, whether specialty incomes are "too high." We discuss this issue in some detail below. The evidence we cite suggests that specialists may earn excessive returns because of limitations on entry into specialties, not because there are too many specialists.[6]

Specialists Drive up Medical Costs. Several recent studies suggest that specialists drive up the cost of medical care. In K. Grumbach and P. Lee's (1991) analysis, the effect of a shift in the proportion of generalists to specialists is expressed by the following equation:

$$\text{total physician income} =$$
$$\text{no. of physicians} \times \text{mean gross income per physician.[7]}$$

Total physician income is computed by using existing income figures and adjusting the ratio of generalists to specialists from current to "desired" levels. This model ignores possible changes in income and other cost implications of changes in physician supply, for example as a result of a change in the way care is delivered.

Other recent articles in medical journals claim that specialists are associated with more costly practice styles. In a review of this literature, P. Franks, C. Clancy, and P. Nutting (1992) report that specialists are associated with higher intensity of care, including the increased use of sophisticated diagnostic technology.[8] Findings such as these cannot be separated from the more general issue of the growing demand for high-tech medicine. Franks, Clancy, and Nutting argue that specialists drive the demand for high-tech medicine. As we will elaborate on below, specialists may be viewed as a response to the demand for this kind of care. The elimination of specialty designations offers no reassurance that this type of care will not be sought out and provided anyway.

Specialists Do Not Provide Higher Quality. Other critics of specialists claim that the quality of care they provide is no higher than the quality provided by generalists. The best evidence against this claim is provided by Harold Luft et al. (1987), who find a significant positive relationship between volume of surgical care and outcomes.[9] In a similar vein, R. Zeiger et al. (1991) find that patients who see specialists in asthma therapy have better outcomes, as measured by rates of relapses.[10] Conversely, Franks and S. Eisenger (1986) find that specialists in obstetrics provide no better perinatal outcomes than do family physicians.[11] While we find the Luft et al. evidence to be quite compelling, we conclude that quality is an issue for selected services.

Managed Care Does Not Need Specialists. Of course, the argument that patients visit specialists even though they offer lower quality at higher cost necessarily assumes that patients are poor consumers. Perhaps individual patients do not always make good consumers—they have limited information about relative physician quality, and they are insulated from cost differentials because of insurance. A central feature of managed care, however, is to shift control over what care is purchased from patients to payers. Payers are motivated to hold down costs, because they keep the savings. They may be better able to judge quality as well, since they can use scale economies efficiently to take advantage of data bases, utilization review programs, and other recent developments in health care information technology.

Studies of managed care organizations show that they reduce the use of inpatient hospital services, presumably with a concomitant reduction in the use of hospital-based specialists.[12] It may be argued that lower use of specialists by managed care organizations is at least in part a product of selectivity, both in terms of the health needs of patients who select such organizations, particularly health maintenance organizations (HMOs), and of their preferences for care. But evidence suggesting that use of specialists is lower under managed care is nevertheless striking, because it implies that when the way care is purchased changes, so does the use of specialists. To the extent one believes there is inappropriate use of specialists in the U.S. health care system, this finding offers a strong argument for focusing on reforms that alter the way care is purchased, rather than imposing direct restrictions on supply.

Specialization as a Sign of a Strong, Productive Economy

In order to judge adequately claims that the market is providing us with too many specialists, it is essential to understand how that market works. The phenomenon of specialization in production has been well understood ever since Adam Smith's description of a pin factory in *The Nature and Causes of the Wealth of Nations,* first published in 1776.[13] Smith noted that when demand for pins was high, the pin factory owner could hire several workers. Each worker would then specialize in a different part of the production process. Consumers benefited from such specialization, as each worker could become more skillful and productive at his or her particular task, and pin quality would increase and production costs fall accordingly.

Smith summarized the relationship between market demand and specialization with the famous dictum, "The division of labor is limited by the extent of the market." "The division of labor" refers to the specialization of the labor force. Specialization is pervasive in labor markets. Lawyers, for example, usually possess specialized knowledge of specific fields—taxation, real estate, antitrust. This specialization allows them to analyze issues intelligently and productively and to formulate arguments in their areas of skill. Specialization is common in engineering, academia, and household repairs (in refrigeration, plumbing, and home electronics, for example). Specialization in medicine is not limited to physicians. Clinical nurse specialists, certified nurse anesthetists, and pediatric nurse practitioners are examples of nurse specialists. Ironically, nurse specialists often claim they are more cost effective than physician specialists providing similar services.[14]

The division of labor is "limited by the extent of the market" because if market demands are insufficient, workers will be unable to justify the time and effort necessary to develop skill in a narrow area of production. Although there are several lawyers in Fairbanks, Alaska, for instance, none are likely to specialize in antitrust issues in health care—the demand for such specialization in Fairbanks is too low.

The extent of the market may increase for a number of reasons. The number of consumers may increase in a market. The wealth of consumers may increase, for example, through improvements in productive efficiency. Finally, the price of complementary products may fall, or the quality may increase. The last reason is especially important in medicine, where technological breakthroughs in diagnosis and treatment have vastly expanded the demand for physicians who can provide them.

Smith's dictum has two important implications. First, specialization is a good thing. It is associated with deepening skill and superior quality. It may also lower costs. Thus, specialists are likely to arrive at the correct solutions to problems sooner than generalists, and their efforts are likely to be of higher quality, lasting longer, with fewer defects. Second, specialization will occur in all growing economies and will in turn help sustain even greater growth.

As economies grow, consumers can afford to support the extra training required by specialists, and they prefer to consume the higher value products they produce. As the late business historian Alfred Chandler noted, specialization engendered by growth may, in turn, foster even greater growth.[15] Chandler observed that specialization of both labor and production processes has sustained economic growth in the United States since the middle of the nineteenth century. At first, the specialists were industrial giants such as du Pont and U.S. Steel, exploiting newly developed productive skills to produce large quantities with high quality and low costs. As our economy has grown, specialists have become more refined. Today's specialists in chemical production may produce pharmaceutical products that target killer diseases. Today's specialists in steel use computerized production technologies to tailor-make products at higher levels of quality than ever before imagined. Economic growth will continue to foster specialization in all aspects of our economy, which in turn will foster greater growth.

The Division of Labor in Medicine. These implications of specialization are just as applicable to medicine as to any other field. Consider the first implication—that specialization improves quality. The past decades have seen many technological advances in diagnosis and treatment. Patients, desiring the benefits of these technologies, demand physicians who possess the special skills needed to take advantage of them. The investments required to master all these skills make it prohibitively costly for a physician to deepen his or her skill in all but a few of them. Specialization is thus a natural outgrowth of the demand for new diagnoses and treatment.

With the growth of technology, we have seen physicians specialize in increasingly narrow areas. Thus, some physicians specialize in thoracic surgery, others in reading diagnostic neuroimages of the brain. Consistent with Smith's predictions, evidence supports the argument that physicians who specialize in a narrow area of medicine have superior skill. Harold Luft and his colleagues at the University of California, San Francisco, have shown that medical providers who do a large number of a specific surgical procedure have far superior outcomes to those providers who do small numbers of one or several procedures. Luft et al. (1987) report, for example, that providers who perform more than 200 open-heart surgeries per year have mortality rates that are one-third that of providers who perform fewer than 25 such surgeries per year, controlling for patient severity.[16]

The second implication of Smith's argument—that growing demand fuels specialization—is also valid in health care. As the world's population demands better treatments for a wider array of diseases, the medical Research and Development sector has produced ever more sophisticated technologies, each of which requires specialized training for implementation. An abbreviated list of recent innovations in diagnosis and treatment includes magnetic resonance imaging, balloon angioplasty, laparoscopic surgery, bone marrow transplantation, liver transplantation, microvascular surgery, and laser surgery.

Even in the absence of technological change, demand and specialization are linked. A decade ago, the RAND Corporation conducted research to determine whether the so-called maldistribution of physicians in the United States represented a market failure (and therefore justified such government interventions as that by the National Health Services Corps). The report by J. Newhouse et al. (1982) demonstrated that Adam Smith's logic was entirely appropriate to understanding the diffusion of primary care and specialty physicians across the United States.[17] Newhouse et al. were able to identify threshold population sizes below which physicians in different specialty groups were unlikely to be found. The smallest thresholds were found for generalists, who could treat a wide range of diseases and therefore could be supported by a relatively small population. As a community grows in size, it becomes more attractive to specialists who require a larger population base to provide enough patients. Perhaps the most significant finding of Newhouse et al. is that as a town's population increases and specialists enter, the generalists tend to leave. This is consistent with the view that consumers prefer the services of specialists to generalists. The continued growth in the number of specialists in small towns and big cities alike is a simple reflection of consumer preferences.

Can the Market Go Wrong?

We have argued that specialization is the natural outcome of a growing market for medical care, stimulated by a combination of rising income and population and technological change. We have also argued that specialization can yield enormous gains in terms of reducing costs or increasing the quality of services. The typical response to the argument is that market forces do not work in health care, and they lead to an overuse of specialists, with costs that offset many of the benefits. S. Schroeder (1992), for instance, cites the "overuse of costly procedures" in the United States.[18] Schroeder and others do not believe that American consumers are buying the correct medical services. Inappropriate consumption may arise for a number of reasons:

1. Specialists may "induce demand" for unnecessary services to boost their incomes.
2. Even in the absence of selfish motives, specialists may provide incorrect information about the best course of treatment.
3. Health insurance may artificially boost demand for all medical ser-

vices because of consumer moral hazard—the susceptibility of consumers to purchasing care whose costs exceed benefits.

We address each of these concerns in turn.

Demand Inducement. More than thirty years ago, Milton Roemer argued that hospitals did not obey the laws of supply and demand. He claimed that hospitals did not have to lose revenues when competitors entered the market, because they could *induce* demand for their services. It is difficult to find anyone today who subscribes to the notion that hospitals can fill their beds willy-nilly without regard for underlying demand. But the underlying notion of supplier-induced demand is very much alive in the case of physician services.

There are two empirical predictions made by inducement theorists. The first is relatively uncontroversial: incentives matter, and providers paid on a fee-for-service basis will provide more services than providers who are capitated. This argument has a solid economic basis and, indeed, substantial evidence to support it. The RAND National Health Insurance Experiment study, for example, found that patients in HMOs that pay their medical staff in salaries are far less likely to be hospitalized than patients in traditional fee-for-service settings.[19]

The second empirical prediction is of greater importance to the debate about specialty quotas: as the supply of physicians increases, they will exploit their dual roles as expert diagnosticians and providers of service, to create demand for their own services. If this is correct, then we may expect ever-increasing numbers of questionable tests and procedures as the supply of specialists grows. There is limited theoretical justification for the link between manpower supply and the amount of inducement. One can obtain limited amounts of such inducement in models that make specific assumptions about the "curvature" of physician "utility functions."[20]

A number of well-known papers purport to show an empirical link between manpower supply and inducement, but these papers are highly controversial. Fuchs (1978) and Cromwell and Mitchell (1986) offer evidence that seems to show, consistent with inducement theory, that the demand curve for physician services is shifted out in those markets with more physicians.[21] The more recent Cromwell and Mitchell estimate suggests that a doubling of the supply of physicians would cause only about a 10 percent increase in demand, however. Even this limited finding is subject to considerable doubt. Auster and Oaxaca (1981), Phelps (1986), and others question the ability of researchers to separate exogenous demand effects from endogenous demand shifting, concluding that the results of Fuchs, Cromwell and Mitchell, and others are biased.[22] Escarce (1992) suggests that so-called inducement is really an access phenomenon—patients in communities that have a surplus of physicians face shorter commutes and shorter waiting times, leading to greater use.[23]

David Dranove and Paul Wehner (1994) suggest that the statistical methods used by V. Fuchs and J. Cromwell and J. Mitchell are faulty.[24] They apply those methods to show that obstetricians induce parents to have children. The absurdity of this finding leads them to question all results based on this method.

If We Cap Specialized Physicians, Why Not Cap Specialized Lawyers?
Suppose, even in the absence of credible evidence, that we accept the argument that a growing supply of specialists will cause patients inappropriately to purchase costly medical services that they otherwise would not have purchased. Could this be a justification for reducing the supply of specialists? If so, the ramifications for other professional services are extraordinary. After all, the problem of the expert-client relationship is common to a wide range of services, such as auto repairs, plumbing, and law. An expert in real estate law, for example, has a financial incentive to tell a client that a real estate contract offers inadequate protection against some unspecified problem. This will cause the client to ask the lawyer to draft the "necessary" clause, thereby driving up the lawyer's fees. If one can justify a cap on the number of medical specialists on the grounds that they can drive up the use of their services, then one can equally well justify a cap on specialized lawyers. We can extend this logic to justify a cap on all specialized labor that provides both special skills and service. An appeal to public safety would not justify special treatment of medicine, since the inducement debate has always been about cost and not quality.

Suppose, carrying this argument further, we believe that all experts induce the overconsumption of their services. Is this sufficient to justify a cap on all expert labor? A simpler solution would be to sever the financial link that purportedly causes the expert to recommend overly expensive services. This is the strategy adopted by many managed care organizations. These organizations pay physicians on a capitated basis, so that the physicians receive a fixed fee per patient regardless of the level of service they provide. If specialists are providing unnecessary services just to boost their incomes, capitation will end the practice.

Another way to reduce the alleged abuses of experts is to have other experts scrutinize their recommendations. Managed care organizations have been quick to follow this strategy as well, through what has come to be known as utilization review. The recommendations of specialists to order tests, admit patients, and perform invasive procedures are scrutinized by utilization review service firms, which then direct providers to the most cost-effective treatment modalities.

Managed care organizations are proliferating in the market. An estimated 90 million Americans are enrolled in HMOs or preferred provider organizations (PPOs) that use managed care principles of capitation, utilization review, or both.[25] The demand for more primary care providers and fewer specialists may be traced to the success of managed care organizations in restructuring the delivery of care. The president's health care plan, if enacted, will accelerate the growth of managed care and therefore accelerate the decline of specialists.

If proponents of caps on specialist training claim that there will still be "too many specialists" and are concerned about issues of inducement, they do not believe that managed care will succeed in rationalizing the provision of care. Managed care is a central feature of the Clinton plan. The call by the Clinton administration for a specialty quota seems to be at odds with its claims that managed care will reduce health care costs. If managed care works, then the Clinton plan will succeed without a specialty quota. If managed care fails to contain costs, the specialty quota is unlikely to be a successful remedy.

Specialists Have Poor Information. Proponents of caps on specialty training may argue that even if incentives are fixed, specialists still make inefficient decisions. By dint of training, they perceive all problems as requiring their specialized training. They may not recognize the interplay of organ systems and may not care about the side effects of their treatments. On balance, the superior skill with which the specialist performs his or her own narrow activity is offset by the costs associated with these shortcomings.

While these complaints may be valid, they cannot justify a cap on specialty training without two additional unstated assumptions. The first is, not only do specialists possess all these bad qualities, but consumers do not realize it, and they therefore continue to be duped into visiting specialists who provide a total quality of care inferior to generalists'. As new technologies of limited or no value are introduced, consumers demand them and the specialists required to provide them. The second is, payers also do not understand what is happening, and they continue to support organizational structures in which consumers have unfettered use of specialists.

The argument that we need to protect consumers from their own ignorance is not new to health care. The managed care revolution, however, has gone a long way to destroy the basis for this argument. Purchasing power increasingly rests with well-informed and financially motivated employers and managed care organizations, who have the power to direct patients to cost effective providers.[26] If specialists continue to practice inefficient medicine under managed care, then again the concept of managed care—the cornerstone of Clinton's health plan—must be challenged.

Consumer Moral Hazard. Most Americans are well insured against the costs of medical care, especially where inpatient services and expensive technologies are involved. Insurance, of course, artificially inflates demand, as the patient and physician may join together in purchasing care whose costs exceed the benefits. This effect applies to all health care services covered by insurance. Standard economic models predict it will be worse for services with more elastic demand, such as preventive care, and for services with more extensive insurance coverage, such as inpatient care. On balance, it is not clear whether moral hazard has a disproportionate effect on specialty care versus primary care.

Specialists versus Specialization

Most of the discussions about specialization in medicine are couched in terms of medical "specialties"—those physicians whose competence in a given area of medicine is affirmed by the credential of a medical specialty organization. Operating under the oversight of the American Board of Medical Specialties and the American Medical Association (AMA), there are some twenty-four recognized medical specialties and more than eighty recognized subspecialties in the United States.[27]

Specialty membership provides an indicator of specialization in the Smithian sense. But it is by no means a perfect one. Smithian specialization implies that workers perform a very narrow set of tasks but possess deep skills that permit them to perform those tasks very effectively. Members of some specialty groups, such as surgical subspecialties and psychiatrists, do engage in narrow sets of tasks. Otolaryngologists, cardiologists, and general surgeons, however, often engage in a wide range of activities.[28] As a consequence, there is often much overlap in the tasks performed by members of different specialties. The boundary lines between specialties, and between specialists and generalists, are not always distinct. At the same time, there is Smithian specialization among physicians with a specific specialty designation. Thus, physicians in family medicine, internal medicine, and general surgery may specialize in particular areas of practice without necessarily obtaining a further specialty designation. Consistent with Smith's notion that specialization increases with the extent of the market, J. Baumgardner (1988) finds that the range of tasks performed by general internists and general surgeons narrows the larger the population center in which they are located.[29]

It is evident from this discussion that specialists may not always be that specialized. Conversely, specialization may occur without specialty designation. This is not unique to medicine. A good example is provided by the legal profession, whose members are often highly specialized but do not generally obtain formal specialty designations. This raises a fundamental issue: is the policy problem in the debate over specialization one of fragmentation in medicine into specialty designations and specialization as an organizational phenomenon, or one of specialization in the division of labor?

The primary justification for ever greater organizational fragmentation of medicine in specialties and subspecialties has been informational. The underlying argument is that it is difficult for consumers to recognize competence on the job. Formal training and the ability to satisfy rigorous specialty board examinations provide consumers with an alternative indicator of ability. Certifying physicians on the basis of training and exams could give consumers and other physicians a low-cost means of evaluating quality.

There are also obvious strategic reasons for the existence of specialty organizations. They may serve as useful vehicles for lobbying on behalf of their members, for exchanging economic as well as technical information, and for bargaining. Thus, specialty organizations have been at the center of national frays over physician payment reform. At the hospital level, specialty departments routinely negotiate with hospital administrations over a broad range of issues.

It is clear, however, that while specialty organizations may serve useful strategic functions, their underlying logic is technological. "Specialties" have not emerged simply as clubs of randomly selected physicians. The glue that typically holds specialty organizations together is the common interests associated with performing similar tasks. And what makes specialty membership truly valuable to most physicians is its role as a market signal.

Individual consumers, providers, and public and private payers alike look to specialty designation as an indicator of quality. Technological advances and accompanying market patterns of specialization render it essential for consumers to have knowledge about who possesses the training necessary to deliver the new technologies. Market demands for specialty designation often win out over resistance by organized medicine. In the early part of this century, for example, the AMA opposed the emergence of radiology as a technical specialty. Instead, the AMA argued that radiology should be viewed as an adjunct to the practice of internal medicine. The marketplace thought otherwise, however. By the early 1920s a growing number of physicians were specializing in X-ray imaging, and in 1925 radiologists were able to win AMA recognition of radiology as a technical specialty.[30]

Today, specialty certification is a widely accepted indicator of competence. It is routine, for instance, for hospitals to require specialty board certification as a condition for membership in specialty departments. Indeed, hospital accreditation standards require at least a minimum number of certified medical personnel, for example, in areas like radiology and pathology. Specialty designation and training also play a central role in determining reimbursement. The Medicare RBRVS (resource-based relative value scale) is an example.

The proliferation of specialty organizations may, of course, make specialization more attractive. Indeed, it would be surprising if it did not. If evaluation of competence is a major problem with using specialists and the emergence of certification systems reduces it, one would expect certification to increase demand and hence specialization. From an efficiency perspective, however, there is nothing automatically bad about this. On the contrary, if the impact of certification is simply to help solve market failure problems associated with imperfect information, standard economic models predict the effect will be to increase efficiency and consumer welfare.

Whether or not providers are permitted to obtain specialty designations, the growth of the market and the emergence of new technologies will feed the demand for physicians with specialized training. Cutting back or eliminating specialty certification will create informational problems for consumers and reduce consumer welfare. These problems may be especially critical for new medical technologies. If physicians are unable to obtain appropriate training, new technologies may go unused, or worse, may be used by untrained physicians. This may reduce the marketability of new technologies, which in turn would reduce the incentives of the R&D sector to develop them. The bottom line is that specialty training and technological change go hand in hand, and it is unwise to advance policy that addresses the training without regard to technological change.

The Troubling History of Federal Medical Manpower Legislation

At a recent conference, one speaker stated that the United States would never be able to train enough primary care practitioners in his lifetime. This reminds us of a claim made in a 1965 report to the American Association of Medical Colleges, funded by the Commonwealth Foundation, that it was "not likely that America will ever be able to produce all the physicians that the nation would like to have."[31] The history of events that led up to this claim and the troubling legacy of the legislative response are highly instructive as to the dangers of federal health manpower programs.

From the end of World War II until 1960, the ratio of physicians to population in the United States held steady at about 141 to 100,000. Around 1960, a series of commissions reported that the United States would have great difficulty maintaining this ratio and that the desired ratio might even be higher. These commissions called for federal action to shore up the supply of physicians in the United States.

The federal government historically has not had a major role in determining the supply of physicians. But in the early 1960s, appealing to concerns about public health, it took a number of steps to increase the supply of physicians.[32] The 1963 Health Professions Education Assistance Act provided more than $800 million to construct new medical schools and to expand existing ones. This amounted to about 13 percent of the total funds spent on medical school construction during the life of the program. The 1968 Health Manpower Act provided loans and scholarships to medical school students and direct capitated subsidies to medical schools. To receive capitation, schools had to expand enrollments by at least 2.5 percent annually. Capitation grants totaled nearly $800 million over the life of the program. In contrast, tuition receipts over this period amounted to $1.8 billion. Thus, capitation amounted to a 30 percent tuition subsidy.

At the same time that funding for domestic medical education increased, restrictions on immigration by foreign medical graduates (FMGs) were eased. Quotas that restricted Asian immigrants were lifted in 1968. A special quota for individuals with "exceptional ability" was created, and physicians were permitted to apply under this criterion. The percentage of new U.S. medical licenses going to FMGs rose from 17 percent in the late 1960s to a peak of 45 percent in 1972, and then it dropped sharply after concerns about the large influx of FMGs led to changes tightening entry rules in 1976.

Direct subsidies to medical schools disappeared by 1980. But the federal government still subsidizes medical education and residency training through its reimbursements to teaching hospitals that care for Medicare patients. We will discuss these subsidies, and why they should be eliminated, later in this monograph.

Programs in the 1960s and 1970s to expand physician supply were all too successful. In 1974, Charles Edwards, assistant secretary of the Department of Health, Education, and Welfare, concluded that the "long perceived physician shortage might soon give way to a physician surplus."[33] By 1980, when the physician-to-population ratio had increased to 197 per 100,000, Secretary Richard Schweiker announced that "the goal of adequacy in medical manpower had been reached." This was an astonishing accomplishment, since it was only sixteen years after the Coggeshall report doubted that goal ever could be reached.

The manpower planners did not believe they had succeeded, however. They looked to a future not of manpower shortage, but of manpower surplus. Thanks to federal support, enrollments in U.S. medical schools had surpassed 64,000, and the number of new physicians entering the profession greatly exceeded the number retiring. In 1980, the Graduate Medical Education National Advisory Council (GMENAC) reported that by the year 1990 there would be a "surplus" of 90,000 physicians, or about 20 percent of the total.[34] Although the current regulatory climate focuses on surpluses of specialists, GMENAC felt that the supply of generalists and specialists were in relative balance and projected surpluses in certain areas of primary care. GMENAC forecast a surplus of 5,000 pediatricians by 1990, for example, and the American Academy of Pediatrics forecast an even larger surplus.[35]

Today, the ratio of physicians to population is around 260 per 100,000, or about 30 percent more than what GMENAC deemed necessary. Using methods similar to those that guided manpower planning efforts in the 1960s through the 1990s, "experts" now forecast surpluses of specialists and shortages of generalists. D. Kindig et al. (1993) estimate that even if the Clinton specialty caps are implemented, we will not have enough primary care physicians to meet anticipated "need" until the year 2040.[36] They support the Clinton initiatives, but they wonder if these will go far enough.

Simple supply and demand helps to explain what went wrong with the federal planning efforts of the past and why new planning efforts should not be implemented now. To understand where the planners went wrong, we need to recognize that the supply of physicians in general, and of specialists in particular, results from a peculiar combination of market forces and professional self-regulation.

Market forces create the demand for medical education. As the attractiveness of the medical profession grows, more undergraduates seek to pursue medicine as a career. There is overwhelming evidence that potential doctors do, indeed, weigh income potential when choosing a career in medicine. M. Noether (1986a) found that after the enactment of Medicare and Medicaid in 1965, the returns to becoming a physician increased dramatically.[37] As a result, applications to medical school increased by about 30 percent by 1975. Between 1976 and 1985, the returns to becoming a physician fell by 14 percent, and applications fell by 30 percent.

Noether also reports that the returns to becoming a physician were only slightly higher than the average return to a college education. This is consistent with the notion that market forces guide the demand for medical education. Economic theory predicts that if college graduates place an important weight on income when choosing careers, then the returns from different career choices will be equilibrated. If not, then those careers with greater returns will attract more graduates, driving down the returns in those careers. Considering that physicians are generally in the top third of their college graduating classes, the fact that they earn slightly higher returns than other college graduates is consistent with an efficient market for medical education.

When medical school applications increase, schools must decide whether to expand. A major obstacle to expansion—finding a pool of qualified applicants—is obviously removed as applications increase. But other obstacles remain. To the extent that the federal government subsidizes education, either directly through capitation programs and grants, or indirectly through Medicare payments, incentives to adjust the number of slots are blunted. A second obstacle to expansion results from professional self-regulation. Many writers have suggested that the American Medical Association effectively controls the U.S. supply of physicians through its influence on accreditation of medical schools.[38] The AMA, acting in behalf of its members, may wish to restrict supply to boost the incomes of those in practice. Entry may be especially restricted for specialties, which control the accreditation of residency training programs.[39] If so, then there are probably fewer specialists than the market will support.

Some evidence that the market would support more specialists than are currently available is provided by W. Mardor and R. Willke (1991), who show that surgical subspecialists, ophthalmologists, radiologists, and anesthesiologists have far higher net discounted earnings than have family practitioners and internists.[40] Additional evidence comes from the residency match program. Although many specialties are fully matched—that is, demand exceeds the number of slots—programs in family practice, internal medicine, and pediatrics are able to fill only about 60 percent of available slots.[41]

Noether (1986b) examined whether the increase in demand for medical education that followed the enactment of Medicare and Medicaid led to a relaxation of entry restrictions by medical schools.[42] She found that between 1965 and 1981, increases in medical school enrollments and FMG immigration resulted in about 120,000 additional physicians practicing in the United States. Of this total, about half the increase was attributable to federal subsidies to medical schools and relaxed immigration laws, and half to medical schools, having opened up new slots to meet the growing demand for medical education. In other words, market forces resulted in a significant increase in physician supply, and they probably would have eliminated the so-called physician shortage.[43] The "excess" supply of physicians that many believe we currently face is an effect of government programs, which magnified the market forces already in place.

Once again, planners believe there are serious problems with medical manpower in the United States. This time, planners have refined their complaints—rather than claiming we have too few or too many physicians, they claim we have too few generalists and too many specialists. Planners do not believe that market forces can effect the desired changes, and so once again they call on the federal government to regulate manpower supply.

The irony of calling for federal manpower training regulation to "fix a problem" allegedly caused by previous federal manpower training regulations is not lost on us. If the current proposals are as "successful" as those of the 1960s and 1970s, we may expect a surplus of generalists within a decade. There will be calls for further manpower planning and turf wars between generalists and nonmedical providers. There may also be a radical shift toward noncredentialed providers using new and sophisticated technologies, as we discuss in the next section. Before that, we turn our attention to one portion of the Clinton quota proposal that will radically change the oversight of medical education.

Allocation of Residency Spots by the National Council of Graduate Medical Education (NCGME). If the Clinton quota plan is enacted as written, the NCGME, an appointed body within the executive branch of the federal government, will have complete control over the allocation of residency training spots in the United States. According to section 3013 of the Clinton plan, the NCGME will allocate residency training spots based on the following criteria: (1) geographic diversity; (2) ethnic and racial diversity; and (3) the recommendations of private organizations.

Under the Clinton plan, the NCGME will have the power to reduce or shut down programs completely. Indeed, if the specialty cap is implemented, the NCGME will be mandated to do so on a grand scale. Given the mandate to achieve geographic, ethnic, and racial diversity, the council will be forced to balance medical and nonmedical criteria. This opens the door to subjectivity and political influence, raising the concern that the NCGME may use its powers to pick and choose among programs for reasons that have more to do with politics than with the quality of the training they provide. Pork-barrel politics and contentious issues such as abortion and fetal tissue research could play significant and unwelcome roles in the allocation of residency slots. One way to mediate some of these problems is to adopt the model developed for military base closings. In this model, an independent commission recommends a list of programs to be cut or closed, and Congress has to approve or disapprove the entire list, rather than vote on individual programs. Even this model may be influenced by politics, however.

Future Risks—Specialization, Quality, and Technological Change

In the past, growing specialization in American medicine has been closely linked with technological change and the rapid adoption of new diagnostic and therapeutic techniques. Patterns of technological change are also likely to play a major role in determining future trends in specialization. S. Schroeder and L. Sandby (1993) and others have argued that specialists themselves have been a driving force in the diffusion of new technology.[44] As we have discussed, however, it is important to distinguish between cause and effect. Specialists clearly have played a central role in implementing the use of new technologies in the U.S. health care delivery system. But this is not the same as creating an underlying demand. Key factors helping to fuel increased high tech care in our system include powerful consumer expectations, massive public subsidies of biomedical research, and demands associated with delegation of purchasing decisions to well-insured individual patients and their doctors.

In the absence of changes in the way we purchase care or finance and organize biomedical research, caps on specialty training programs are unlikely to have much effect on the underlying style of practice in U.S. medicine. Rather, they are likely to lead to a reorganization in the way high-technology services are provided. Conversely, changes in the way care is purchased, which in fact are already occurring, or in the organization of biomedical research could have dramatic implications for the style of medical practice. The extent to which specialty caps might impose binding constraints on the organization of care in this case is unclear.

More rigorous standards for the use of new technologies will not necessarily lead to decreases in demand for specialists.

As a starting point for examining the future, consider possible trends in specialization and the effect of specialty caps if, unrealistically, no changes occur in the way care is purchased or the way biomedical research is funded and organized. In the absence of any checks on demand or availability of new, technologically oriented services, pressures will almost certainly continue for increased specialization in medicine. To the extent that specialists have provided the primary routes for access to these technologies, caps could lead to bottlenecks in the short run. In the long run, if underlying demand remains strong for new services, then either (1) the government will have to place explicit quotas on access to new services, or (2) health care delivery will replicate the existing style of U.S. medical practice while reducing reliance on formally trained specialists.

Thus, we could find it increasingly difficult to get an appointment with a specialist graduate of an approved program. And if we do get an appointment, it could be even more expensive than it is today. If caps lead to shortages of specialists at existing prices, in the absence of price controls large windfall profits could arise for those lucky enough to gain entry into specialty programs. This does not mean that instead we will receive all our care from a "gatekeeper" physician—that is, one acting as our primary contact point with the health care system. Nor does it mean that the care that gatekeepers provide will necessarily be low-tech.

When a serious problem develops, if a specialist is unavailable or very costly, there will be strong pressures on efficiency grounds to refer to a generalist who has particular knowledge of the problem at hand. If we have a heart problem, for example, and caps limit the availability of cardiologists, we will probably be referred to a general internist who treats primarily cardiovascular patients but who has no formal credentials, and whose qualifications are more difficult to evaluate. Moreover, to the extent that caps make referrals more difficult, there will be strong incentives to render new technologies more accessible to generalists. This may ease the demand for specialists and for specialized skills. But it will not necessarily lead to the most cost-effective provision of services, and it may compromise quality— for example, a complex diagnostic test interpreted by a generalist may not lead to cost-effective decision making.

The scenario described above assumes no change in either the demand side of the market for health care or the behavior of the biomedical research enterprise. Dramatic changes, of course, have already begun in the way care is purchased with the recent rapid growth of managed care, and the Clinton proposals for managed competition would accelerate these changes. The underlying notion in managed care is that by shifting the locus of purchasing decisions away from patients and toward centralized payer organizations, we can rationalize purchasing, achieve greater "value for money," and move away from the indiscriminate use of expensive technologies whose costs exceed any benefits they yield.

The word "indiscriminate" is key here. Implicit in much of the debate over specialists is the presumption that better value for money implies greater reliance on primary care. If this is true and managed care accomplishes its mission and leads to major shifts in purchasing patterns away from high-tech medicine toward primary care, caps on specialty training could end up being largely irrelevant. Just as the number of training slots for primary care currently exceeds demand and many specialty programs are oversubscribed, the reverse could soon be the case, as the market for specialty services begins to dry up.

It is important to point out, however, that there is no a priori reason why more primary care per se is synonymous with greater value for money in medicine. At least in some areas, it may turn out that *more* reliance on specialists, but in a more discriminating fashion regarding the services they provide, is the most effective means of delivering care given the cost-quality trade-offs of purchasers. In this case, specialty caps could result in serious shortages if federal planners misjudge demand across the board or in particular areas of medicine. Given the history of federal manpower legislation, such misjudgments are to be expected. As a result, managed care organizations could be left with the choice of using less specialty services than they would like or attempting to substitute generalists for specialists where quality may be hard to evaluate.

Similar issues exist regarding rationalization of the supply of new technology and biomedical research. In many discussions of specialization, the availability of new medical technologies is treated as exogenous, an independent force for change. It is possible, however, that changes in the way care is purchased may significantly affect the directions of research. Indeed, as discussed by Baumgardner (1991), changes in reimbursement such as the introduction of the Medicare Prospective Payment System may already have begun to do so, although the long lags that may be involved make this difficult to determine.[45] In any case, there has been a major growth in efforts to develop tools for evaluating medical outcomes and comparing the efficiency of treatments and their costs. And as B. Weisbrod (1991) points out, potential cost effectiveness could become one of the criteria used in allocating public subsidies for research, reinforcing changes taking place on the demand side of health care markets.[46] This could result in the more prudent introduction of new technology. But once again, the implications for use of specialists are not obvious, and caps could create problems.

What Should Congress Do?

The federal government has had a major role in causing the current climate of crisis surrounding specialization. Federal action is clearly an important part of any solution. The government need not rely significantly on quotas to influence appropriately the flow of physicians into specialties. The government should direct its attention to the following areas of action: subsidization of medical education and residency training; regulations governing the use and geographic mobility of health personnel; and policies regarding funding of medical research.

Subsidization of Medical Education and Residency Training. Although construction grants and capitation for medical schools are no longer important, subsidies for specialty training remain significant. The most important subsidies arise through Medicare payments for hospital services. Medicare makes a "direct" payment based on the number of full-time equivalent residents employed by each hospital. The Council of Graduate Medical Education estimates that the direct payment for physician training will amount to $1.5 billion in fiscal year 1994.[47] In addition, Medicare marks up its diagnostic related group (DRG) payments to teaching hospitals according to the indirect medical education factor. This factor is based on the ratio of residents to hospital beds and is currently 7 percent for each resident per 100 beds. Thus, a hospital with 100 residents and 500 beds receives DRG payments that are 14 percent higher than those of a hospital without residents. The indirect medical education factor accounts for 5.7 percent of total DRG payments,[48] and the Council of Graduate Medical Education estimates that subsidies to residency training through the indirect factor will amount to $4.1 billion in fiscal year 1994.

Teaching hospitals may justify these enormous subsidies by claiming that the training of residents is a public good that should be undertaken by teaching hospitals. Of course, residents provide considerable inpatient care, for which teaching hospitals receive reimbursement. Teaching hospitals might respond that inpatient operating costs are higher when hospitals use residents, and therefore DRG payments should be adjusted to account for the difference.[49] Residents drive up costs for two reasons. First, residents have inefficient practice styles. They order more tests, and they prolong inpatients stays. Second, teaching hospitals may attract sicker patients, and differences in severity may not be taken fully into account by DRGs. Even the Health Care Financing Administration acknowledges that the 7 percent adjustment is overly generous.[50]

Regardless of the specific indirect factor chosen by HCFA, the argument that Medicare should pay more to teaching hospitals because their costs are higher is consistent with a general pattern of subsidizing medical education. The vast majority of the $5.6 billion in subsidies provided through the direct and indirect education factors goes to support the training of specialists.[51] Such subsidies artificially increase the supply of specialists. It is hard to justify the continuance of subsidies if the goal is a reduction in the supply of specialists. If that is the goal, then Medicare should eliminate its direct and indirect subsidies to medical education. An obvious variant of this policy is for Medicare to limit its subsidy to the period required for postgraduate training in primary care. This eliminates market distortions that favor specialty care, and it echoes a recommendation by Ginzberg.[52] Some physicians propose another variant: increase the subsidies to generalist training.[53] This will also increase the relative supply of generalists, but it is a costly way to do so, amounting to a wealth transfer to the medical profession. It will also make medicine a more attractive profession in general, leading to an even larger supply of physicians.

Teaching hospitals will argue that if subsidies end, they will continue to offer specialty training but will have to charge residents for it rather than offer substantial stipends. It is debatable whether this will happen, but if it does, we find nothing inherently troubling about it. This will force specialists-in-training to pay for the costs of their postgraduate education. This reduces the demand for specialty training to the economically appropriate level, without the dangers associated with quotas.

The government should subsidize curriculum development for specialists who wish to develop skills in general practice. Specialists already provide some primary care, and they may do so with good quality.[54] Special curricula will enhance the redeployment of specialists in general care. To the extent that curriculum development is a public good, there is a role for the government to play. More generally (no pun intended), curriculum development at all stages of medical education may lead to changes that encourage more cost-effective styles of practice. It is not clear, however, why the medical profession would not supply these changes itself in response to pressure from managed care.

Payment Reform. As a major purchaser of care, the government is in a position to exert major influence on the mixture of services through the way it pays for care. The resource-based relative value scale (RBRVS) is a controversial example of one attempt to do so. There are studies underway to evaluate the impact of RBRVS on physician incomes and the demand for specialty training. The Clinton proposals for extending managed care to the public sector represent a far more powerful method to affect demand. These demand-side initiatives may be far more effective in achieving desired levels of specialization than is a supply-side quota.

Licensing Regulations. Licensure may further inflate the demand for specialists in two ways. First, it limits the ability to substitute nonmedical personnel for physicians. Second, it limits geographic mobility.

The restrictions on the use of physician extenders such as nurse practitioners are well known. Although attention in this area is focused on primary care, it also applies to specialists. Nurse midwives and nurse anesthetists are variously subject to licensure restrictions that may limit their ability to substitute for physicians. Various interest groups have asked Congress to provide antitrust exemptions permitting them to exclude physician extenders even in monopoly markets. Congress should eliminate institutional biases against physician extenders, and continue vigorously to enforce antitrust laws that enable physician extenders to compete fairly with monopoly physician providers. Specialty certifications, although not a form of licensure, also affect the division of labor in important ways because they are frequently used by Medicare in setting payment rates. The resource-based relative value scale, for example, has explicit adjustments to pay for the costs of residency training, but it does not adjust payments for generalists to develop the skills necessary to substitute for specialists. The RBRVS should be adjusted to eliminate subsidies for residency training.

At the same time that licensure restrictions artificially inflate the incomes of specialists, other restrictions reduce the available supply of primary care providers. Clinical nurse specialists, pediatric nurse practitioners, and others still face obstacles to augment significantly the supply of primary care services. Expanding credentialing practices to recognize that non-physician providers may possess the skills necessary to order tests, prescribe drugs, and so forth, and to receive reimbursement for doing so, will go a long way to ensuring an adequate supply of primary care providers.

A less important issue is state licensure laws that restrict mobility of physicians. It seems likely that managed care will lead to substantial redistributions of generalists and specialists. A well-functioning national market for physicians will be desirable from this perspective. Existing state restrictions on physician in-migration will compromise the effectiveness of managed care. States must be encouraged to offer reciprocity to physicians licensed in other states.

Redirect Medical R&D. New technology does not have to be more costly (Weisbrod 1991). Researchers can direct their efforts toward innovations that reduce health care costs, if given the incentive to do so. Specialists would then use their skills to apply cost-reducing technologies, and they would be essential to cost-containment activities.

The National Institute of Health (NIH) is the largest funder of medical research in the United States, with a current budget of approximately $10 billion. Research leading to most new drugs, as well as to many new diagnostic and treatment technologies, was subsidized by the NIH. The NIH should explicitly consider the cost implications of the research programs it supports. The NIH and other government agencies should ask grant applicants to provide an economic impact statement on a voluntary basis and should give greater weight in their budget allocations to those projects offering the greatest promise of containing costs. We are not the first to promote this idea; prominent scientists are increasingly concerned with getting researchers to think in terms of their effect on costs.[55]

Notes

1. David P. Kindig, James M. Cultice, and Fitzhugh Mullan, 1993, "The Elusive Generalist Physician; Can We Reach a 50 Percent Goal?" *New England Journal of Medicine*, vol. 270 (1993), pp. 1069–73.

2. Robert M. Politzer, et al., "Primary Care Physician Supply and the Medically Underserved," *JAMA*, vol. 266, pp. 104–9.

3. Steven A. Schroeder, and Lewis G. Sandy, "Specialty Distribution of U.S. Physicians—The Invisible Driver of Health Care Costs," *New England Journal of Medicine*, vol. 328 (1993), pp. 961–3.

4. William Mardor, and Rich Willke, "Comparisons of the Value of Physician Time by Specialty," in H.E. Frech, ed., *Regulating Doctors' Fees* (Washington, D.C.: AEI Press, 1991).

5. Steven A. Schroeder and Lewis E. Sandy, "Specialty Distribution of U.S. Physicians."

6. For a complete discussion, see David Dranove and Mark Satterthwaite, "The Implications of Resource-Based Relative Value Scale for Physicians' Fees, Incomes, and Specialty Choices," in Frech, *Regulating Doctors' Fees.*

7. Kevin Grumbach and Phillip R. Lee, "How Many Physicians Can We Afford?" *JAMA*, vol. 265 (1991), pp. 2369–72.

8. Peter Franks, Carolyn Clancy, and Paul A. Nutting, "Gatekeeping Revisited—Protecting Patients from Overtreatment," *New England Journal of Medicine*, vol. 327 (1992), pp. 424–29.

9. Harold S. Luft, Sandra S. Hunt and Susan C. Maerki, "The Volume-Outcome Relationship: Practice Makes Perfect or Selective Referral Patterns?" *Health Services Research*, vol. 22 (1987), pp. 157–81.

10. Robert S. Zeiger, et al., "Facilitated Referral to Asthma Specialist Reduces Relapses in Asthma Emergency Room Visits," *Journal of Allergy and Clinical Immunology*, vol. 87 (1991), pp. 1160–68.

11. Peter Franks and Steven Eisenger, "Adverse Perinatal Outcomes: Is Physician Specialty a Risk Factor?" *Journal of Family Practice*, vol. 24 (1987), pp. 152–6.

12. W. Manning, et al., "A Controlled Trial of the Effect of a Prepaid Group Practice on Use of Services," *New England Journal of Medicine*, vol. 310 (1984), pp. 1505–10.

13. Adam Smith, *An Inquiry into the Nature and Causes of the Wealth of Nations* (Homewood, IL.: Richard D. Irwin, 1963).

14. See, for example, Donald Gardner, "The CNS as Cost Manager,"

Clinical Nurse Specialist, vol. 6 (1992), pp. 112–16.

15. Alfred Chandler, *Scale and Scope* (Cambridge, Mass.: Harvard University Press, 1990).

16. Harold S. Luft, Sandra S. Hunt and Susan C. Maerki, "The Volume-Outcome Relationship."

17. Joseph P. Newhouse, Albert P. Williams, Bruce W. Bennett, and William B. Schwartz, "Does the Geographical Distribution of Physicians Reflect Market Failure?" *Bell Journal of Economics,* vol. 13 (1982), pp. 493–505.

18. Steven Schroeder, "Physician Supply and the U.S. Medical Marketplace," *Health Affairs,* vol. 11 (1992), pp. 235–43.

19. Results of the RAND experiment appear in a number of papers. For a good summary see chapter 5 in Charles Phelps, *Health Economics* (New York: Harper Collins, 1992).

20. See, for example, Thomas McGuire and Mark Pauly, "Physician Response to Fee Changes with Multiple Payers," *Journal of Health Economics,* vol. 10 (1991), pp. 385–410.

21. Victor Fuchs, "The Supply of Surgeons and the Demand for Operations," *Journal of Human Resources,* vol. 13 (Supplement) (1978), pp. 35–56. J. Cromwell and Janet Mitchell, "Physician-induced Demand for Surgery," *Journal of Health Economics,* vol. 5 (1986), pp. 293–313.

22. Rich Auster and Rich Oaxaca, "Identification of Supplier-induced Demand in the Health Care Sector" *Journal of Human Resources,* vol. 16 (1981), pp. 327–42. Charles Phelps, "Induced Demand—Can We Ever Know Its Extent?" *Journal of Health Economics,* vol. 5 (1986), pp. 355–65.

23. J. Escarce, "Explaining the Association between the Surgeon Supply and Utilization," *Inquiry,* vol. 29 (1992), pp. 403–415.

24. David Dranove and Paul Wehner, "Physician-Induced Demand for Childbirths," *Journal of Health Economics* (forthcoming).

25. See Employee Benefit Retirement Institute, *Databook on Employee Benefits* (Washington, D.C: EBRI, 1992). While the private sector has embraced managed care, managed care has been all but shut out of the Medicare and Medicaid markets. (Laws do permit Medicare and Medicaid enrollees to select managed care firms, but the laws place many restrictions on providers and enrollees and have been relatively ineffective at expanding managed care enrollments.)

26. For a review of the literature on the emergence of managed care and the effects of shifting the locus of purchasing power from patients to payers, see David Dranove and William White, "Recent Theory and Evidence on Competition in Hospital Markets," *Journal of Economics and Management Strategy,* vol. 3 (forthcoming).

27. Linda Page, "Accreditors Put Brakes on Subspecialty Proliferation," *American Medical News,* vol. 35 (1992), pp. 36–7.

28. James Baumgardner, "What is a Specialist Anyway?" unpublished working paper, Duke University (1992).

29. J. Baumgardner, "Physicians' Services and the Division of Labor Across Local Markets," *Journal of Political Economy*, vol. 96 (1988), pp. 948–82.

30. R. Brecher and E. Brecher, *The Rays: A History of Radiology in the United States and Canada* (Baltimore: Williams & Wilkins, 1969).

31. Lawrence Coggeshall, *Planning for Medical Progress Through Education* (Washington, D.C.: Association of American Medical Colleges, 1965), p. 26.

32. For further details, see Monica Noether, "The Effect of Government Policy Changes on the Supply of Physicians: Expansion of a Competitive Fringe," *Journal of Law and Economics*, vol. 29 (1986), pp. 231–62.

33. For further discussion of events surrounding the expansion of the supply of physicians, see Eli Ginzberg, "Physician Supply Policies and Health Reform," *JAMA*, vol. 268 (1992), pp. 3115–18.

34. "Summary Report of the Graduate Medical Education National Advisory Committee to the Secretary, Department of Health and Human Services," U.S. Department of Health and Human Services, DHHS Publication no. (HRA) 81–651, 1980.

35. See Robert L. Johnson et al., "Pediatric Workforce Statement," *Pediatrics*, vol. 92 (1993), pp. 725–30.

36. David Kindig, James M. Cultice and Fitzhugh Mullan, "The Elusive Generalist Physician; Can We Reach a 50 Percent Goal?" *JAMA*, vol. 270 (1993), pp. 1069–73.

37. Monica Noether, "The Growing Supply of Physicians: Has the Market Become More Competitive?" *Journal of Labor Economics*, vol. 4 (1986), pp. 503–37.

38. See, for example, M. Friedman, "Occupational Licensure," in *Capitalism and Freedom* (Chicago: University of Chicago Press, 1962).

39. See David Dranove and Mark Satterthwaite, "The Implications of Resource-Based Relative Value Scales."

40. William Mardor and Richard Willke, "Comparisons of the Value of Physician Time by Specialty," in Frech, ed., *Regulating Doctors' Fees.*

41. B. Stimmel, "The Crisis in Primary Care and the Role of Medical Schools," *JAMA*, vol. 268 (1992), pp. 2060–65.

42. Monica Noether, "The Effect of Government Policy Changes on the Supply of Physicians: Expansion of a Competitive Fringe," *Journal of Law and Economics*, vol. 29 (1986), pp. 231–62.

43. Political forces may have also played a role, though this is difficult to calculate.

44. Steven A. Schroeder and Lewis G. Sandy, "Specialty Distribution of U.S. Physicians."

45. J. Baumgardner, "The Interaction Between Forms of Insurance Contract and Types of Technical Change in Medical Care," *RAND Journal of Economics*, vol. 22 (1991), pp. 36–53.

46. Burt Weisbrod, "The Health Care Quadrilemma: An essay on Technological Change, Insurance Quality of Care, and Cost Containment," *Journal of Economic Literature*, vol. 29 (1991), pp. 523–52.

47. Council of Graduate Medical Education. *Fourth Report to Congress*, January 1994.

48. Prospective Payment Assessment Commission, *Medicare and the American Health Care System: Report to the Congress*, Washington, D.C., June 1992, pp. 39–40.

49. Federal Register, vol. 57 (108): 23661.

50. *Ibid.*

51. More than 70 percent of new residents in any year are training to be specialists, and specialist training lasts longer than generalist training.

52. Eli Ginzberg, "Physician Supply Policies and Health Reform," *JAMA*, vol. 268 (1992), pp. 3115–8.

53. For a discussion of these options, see Emily Friedman, "Whither Medical Education?" *JAMA*, vol. 270 (1993), pp. 1473–76.

54. Allen J. Dietrich and Harold Goldberg, "Preventive Content of Adult Primary Care: Do Generalists and Subspecialists Differ?" *American Journal of Public Health*, vol. 74 (1984), pp. 223–27.

55. "Can Researchers Help to Lower Costs?" *Science*, vol. 261 (1993), p. 417.

About the Authors

DAVID DRANOVE is associate professor of management and strategy and of health services management at Northwestern University's Kellogg Graduate School of Management. His research activities focus on the health care industry and related industries, and he is on the editorial boards of the *Journal of Health Economics* and the *Journal of Medical Practice Management*.

WILLIAM D. WHITE is an associate professor in the Department of Economics at the University of Illinois at Chicago and associate professor and associate director of the Institute of Government and Public Affairs at the University of Illinois. He is the author of studies on the structure and performance of markets for hospital services, the design of health care payment systems, and the economics of professional regulation. He is a member of the editorial board of the *Journal of Health Politics, Policy and Law*.

AEI Studies in Health Policy

Special Studies in Health Reform